The

Complete Ketogenic

Air Fryer Lunch

Recipe Book

A Set of Mouth-Watering Recipes
for Delicious Ketogenic Air Fryer
Meals

Nolan Turner

advice. The content within this book has been derived from various sources. Please consult a licensed professional before attempting any techniques outlined in this book.

By reading this document, the reader agrees that under no circumstances is the author responsible for any losses, direct or indirect, which are incurred as a result of the use of information contained within this document, including, but not limited to, — errors, omissions, or inaccuracies.

Table of Contents

Radish and Tuna Salad

Prep time: 15 minutes **Cooking time:** 8 minutes **Servings:** 2

Ingredients:

½ cup radish sprouts

8 oz tuna, smoked, boneless and shredded

1 egg, beaten

1 tablespoon coconut flour

½ teaspoon ground coriander

½ teaspoon lemon zest, grated

1 tablespoon olive oil

½ teaspoon salt

1 tablespoon lemon juice

½ cup radish, sliced

Directions:

Mix up the tuna with coconut flour, ground coriander, lemon zest, and egg. Stir the mixture until homogenous. Preheat the air fryer to 400F. Then make the small tuna balls and put them in the hot air fryer. Sprinkle the tuna balls with ½ tablespoon of olive oil. Cook the tuna balls for 8 minutes. Flip the tuna balls on another side after 4 minutes of cooking.

Meanwhile, mix up together radish sprouts and radish. Sprinkle the mixture with remaining olive oil, salt, and lemon juice. Shake it well. Then top the salad with tuna balls.

Nutrition: calories 342, fat 18.9, fiber 1.8, carbs 5.4, protein 35.7

Pork Bowls

Preparation time: 5 minutes **Cooking time**: 20 minutes **Servings:** 4

Ingredients:

½ pound pork stew meat, cubed

¼ cup keto tomato sauce 1 tablespoon olive oil

cups mustard greens

1 yellow bell pepper, chopped 2 green onions, chopped

Salt and black pepper to the taste

Directions:

In a pan that fits your air fryer, mix all the ingredients, toss, introduce the pan in the air fryer and cook at 370 degrees F for 20 minutes. Divide into bowls and serve for lunch.

Nutrition: calories 265, fat 12, fiber 3, carbs 5, protein 14

Broccoli Salad

Prep time: 10 minutes **Cooking time:** 18 minutes **Servings:** 2

Ingredients:

1 cup broccoli florets

1 teaspoon olive oil

1 tablespoon hazelnuts, chopped

4 bacon slices

½ teaspoon salt

½ teaspoon lemon zest, grated

½ teaspoon sesame oil

Directions:

Mix up broccoli florets with olive oil, salt, and lemon zest. Shake the vegetables well. Preheat the air fryer to 385F. Put the broccoli in the air fryer basket and cook for 8 minutes. Shake the broccoli after 4 minutes of cooking. Then transfer the broccoli in the salad bowl. Place the bacon in the air fryer and cook it at 400F for 10 minutes or until it is crunchy. Chop the cooked bacon and add in the broccoli. After this, add hazelnuts and sesame oil. Stir the salad gently.

Nutrition: calories 266, fat 20.9, fiber 1.4, carbs 4.1, protein 15.7

Chicken Stew

Preparation time: 5 minutes **Cooking time**: 30 minutes **Servings:** 6

Ingredients:

tablespoon butter, soft 4 celery stalks, chopped

red bell peppers, chopped

1 pound chicken breasts, skinless, boneless and cubed 2 teaspoons garlic, minced

Salt and black pepper to the taste

½ cup coconut cream

Directions:

Grease a baking dish that fits your air fryer with the butter, add all the ingredients in the pan and toss them. Introduce the dish in the fryer, cook at 360 degrees F for 30 minutes, divide into bowls and serve for lunch.

Nutrition: calories 246, fat 12, fiber 2, carbs 6, protein 12

Chives Chicken

Prep time: 10 minutes **Cooking time:** 12 minutes
Servings: 4

Ingredients:

4 chicken tenders

½ teaspoon ground paprika

½ teaspoon salt

½ cup coconut flakes

1 egg, beaten

1 tablespoon heavy cream

½ teaspoon dried dill

½ teaspoon onion powder

1 tablespoon chives, grinded

1 teaspoon sesame oil

Directions:

Beat the chicken tenders gently with the help of the kitchen hammer. In the mixing bowl mix up salt, eggs heavy cream, cried dill, onion powder, and chives. Then dip the chicken tenders in the egg mixture and coat in the coconut flakes. Repeat the same steps one more time. Preheat the air fryer to 400F. Sprinkle the air fryer basket with sesame oil and place the chicken tenders inside. Cook the rack chicken for 6 minutes. Then flip it on another side and cook for 6 minutes more or until the chicken is light brown.

Nutrition: calories 354, fat 17.8, fiber 1.1, carbs 2.2, protein 44.2

Rosemary Zucchini Mix

Preparation time: 5 minutes **Cooking time**: 12 minutes **Servings:** 4

Ingredients:

¼ cup keto tomato sauce 1 tablespoon olive oil

8 zucchinis, roughly cubed

Salt and black pepper to the taste

¼ teaspoon rosemary, dried

½ teaspoon basil, chopped

Directions:

Grease a pan that fits your air fryer with the oil, add all the ingredients, toss, introduce the pan in the fryer and cook at 350 degrees F for 12 minutes. Divide into bowls and serve for lunch.

Nutrition: calories 200, fat 6, fiber 2, carbs 4, protein 6

Pork Casserole

Prep time: 15 minutes **Cooking time:** 30 minutes **Servings:** 6

Ingredients:

1 teaspoon taco seasonings

1 teaspoon sesame oil

1 teaspoon salt

2 cups ground pork

½ cup keto tomato sauce

2 low carb tortillas

½ cup Cheddar cheese, shredded

¼ cup mozzarella cheese, shredded

Directions:

Chop the tortillas roughly. Brush the air fryer pan with sesame oil and place ½ part of chopped tortilla in it. In the mixing bowl mix up taco seasonings, ground pork, and salt. Place ½ part of ground pork over the tortillas and top it with mozzarella cheese. Then cover the cheese with remaining tortillas, ground pork, and Cheddar cheese. Pour the marinara sauce over the cheese and cover the casserole with foil. Secure the edges. Preheat the air fryer to 395F. Put the casserole in the air fryer and cook it for 20 minutes. Then remove the foil and cook it for 10 minutes more.

Nutrition: calories 404, fat 27, fiber 2.9, carbs 7.4, protein 30.9

Turkey Stew

Preparation time: 5 minutes **Cooking time**: 25 minutes **Servings:** 4

Ingredients:

½ pound brown mushrooms, sliced Salt and black pepper to the taste

¼ cup keto tomato sauce

1 turkey breast, skinless, boneless, cubed and browned 1 tablespoon parsley, chopped

Directions:

In a pan that fits your air fryer, mix the turkey with the mushrooms, salt, pepper and tomato sauce, toss, introduce in the fryer and cook at 350 degrees F for 25 minutes. Divide into bowls and serve for lunch with parsley sprinkled on top.

Nutrition: calories 220, fat 12, fiber 2, carbs 5, protein 12

Lime Cod

Prep time: 8 minutes **Cooking time:** 13 minutes **Servings:** 2

Ingredients:

2 lime slices

1 tablespoon lime juice

1 teaspoon lime zest, grated

¼ teaspoon ground black pepper

1 teaspoon sesame oil

½ teaspoon chili flakes

1-pound cod fillets, boneless

Directions:

Rub the fish with lime zest, ground black pepper, chili flakes, and lime juice. Then brush it with sesame oil. Preheat the air fryer to 400F. Put the cod in the air fryer basket and cook it for 13 minutes. Then cut the cooked fish into halves and top with the sliced lime.

Nutrition: calories 227, fat 4, fiber 0.5, carbs 4.8, protein 42.2

Cayenne Zucchini Mix

Prep time: 20 minutes **Cooking time:** 16 minutes **Servings:** 2

Ingredients:

2 zucchini

½ cup Monterey jack cheese, shredded

¼ cup ground chicken

1 teaspoon salt

½ teaspoon cayenne pepper

1 teaspoon olive oil

Directions:

Trim the zucchini and cut it into the Hasselback. In the mixing bowl mix up ground chicken, cheese, salt, and cayenne pepper. The fill the zucchini with chicken mixture and sprinkle with olive oil. Preheat the air fryer to 400F. Put the Hasselback zucchini in the air fryer and cook for 16 minutes at 400F.

Nutrition: calories 191, fat 12.6, fiber 2.3, carbs 7, protein 14.4

Garlic Pork and Sprouts Stew

Preparation time: 5 minutes **Cooking time**: 25 minutes **Servings:** 4

Ingredients:

2 tablespoons olive oil 2 tomatoes, cubed

2 garlic cloves, minced

½ pound Brussels sprouts, halved 1 pound pork stew meat, cubed

¼ cup veggie stock

¼ cup keto tomato sauce

Salt and black pepper to the taste 1 tablespoon chives, chopped

Directions:

Heat up a pan that fits the air fryer with the oil over medium-high heat, add the meat, garlic, salt and pepper, stir and brown for 5 minutes. Add all the other ingredients except the chives, toss, introduce in the fryer and cook at 380 degrees F for 20 minutes. Divide the stew into bowls and serve with chives sprinkled on top.

Nutrition: calories 200, fat 6, fiber 2, carbs 4, protein 13

Ground Turkey Mix

Preparation time: 5 minutes **Cooking time**: 25 minutes **Servings:** 4

Ingredients:

pound turkey meat, ground

A pinch of salt and black pepper 2 tablespoons olive oil

teaspoons parsley flakes

1 pound green beans, trimmed and halved 2 teaspoons garlic powder

Directions:

Heat up a pan that fits the air fryer with the oil over medium-high heat, add the meat and brown it for 5 minutes. Add the remaining ingredients, toss, put the pan in the machine and cook at 370 degrees F for 20 minutes. Divide between plates and serve.

Nutrition: calories 274, fat 12, fiber 3, carbs 6, protein 15

Basil Mascarpone Chicken Fillets

Prep time: 15 minutes **Cooking time:** 12 minutes **Servings:** 4

Ingredients:

1 tablespoon fresh basil, chopped

4 oz Mozzarella, sliced

12 oz chicken fillet

1 tablespoon nut oil

1 teaspoon chili flakes

1 teaspoon mascarpone

Directions:

Brush the air fryer pan with nut oil. Then cut the chicken fillet on 4 servings and beat them gently with a kitchen hammer. After this, sprinkle the chicken fillets with chili flakes and put in the air fryer pan in one layer. Top the fillets with fresh basil and sprinkle with mascarpone. After this, top the chicken fillets with sliced Mozzarella.

Preheat the air fryer to 375F. Put the pan with Caprese chicken fillets in the air fryer and cook them for 12 minutes.

Nutrition: calories 274, fat 14.9, fiber 0, carbs 1.1, protein 32.8

Turkey with Cabbage

Preparation time: 5 minutes **Cooking time**: 25 minutes **Servings:** 4

Ingredients:

1 pound turkey meat, ground

A pinch of salt and black pepper 2 tablespoons butter, melted

1 ounce chicken stock

1 small red cabbage head, shredded 1 tablespoon sweet paprika, chopped 1 tablespoon parsley, chopped

Directions:

Heat up a pan that fits the air fryer with the butter, add the meat and brown for 5 minutes. Add all the other ingredients, toss, put the pan in the air fryer and cook at 380 degrees F for 20 minutes. Divide everything between plates and serve.

Nutrition: calories 284, fat 13, fiber 4, carbs 5, protein 14

Fried Chicken Halves

Prep time: 20 minutes **Cooking time:** 75 minutes
Servings: 4

Ingredients:

16 oz whole chicken

1 tablespoon dried thyme

1 teaspoon ground cumin

1 teaspoon salt

1 tablespoon avocado oil

Directions:

Cut the chicken into halves and sprinkle it with dried thyme, cumin, and salt. Then brush the chicken halves with avocado oil. Preheat the air fryer to 365F. Put the chicken halves in the air fryer and cook them for 60 minutes. Then flip the chicken halves on another side and cook them for 15 minutes more.

Nutrition: calories 224, fat 9, fiber 0.5, carbs 0.9, protein 33

Cheddar Garlic Turkey

Preparation time: 5 minutes **Cooking time:** 20 minutes **Servings:** 4

Ingredients:

1 big turkey breast, skinless, boneless and cubed Salt and black pepper to the taste

¼ cup cheddar cheese, grated

¼ teaspoon garlic powder 1 tablespoon olive oil

Directions:

Rub the turkey cubes with the oil, season with salt, pepper and garlic powder and dredge in cheddar cheese. Put the turkey bits in your air fryer's basket and cook at 380 degrees F for 20 minutes. Divide between plates and serve with a side salad.

Nutrition: calories 240, fat 11, fiber 2, carbs 5, protein 12

Chicken Bites and Chili Sauce

Prep time: 15 minutes **Cooking time:** 10 minutes **Servings:** 5

Ingredients:

15 oz chicken fillet

1 tablespoon peanut oil

1 teaspoon chili sauce

1 teaspoon lemon zest, grated

½ teaspoon onion powder

1 egg, beaten

½ teaspoon salt

Directions:

Cut the chicken fillet on 5 pieces and sprinkle with chili sauce, lemon zest, onion powder, and salt. Then dip every chicken piece in the beaten egg.

Preheat the air fryer to 400F. Sprinkle the air fryer basket with peanut oil. Put the chicken bites in the air fryer in one layer and cook them for 5 minutes from each side.

Nutrition: calcries 199, fat 9.9, fiber 0, carbs 0.4, protein 25.7

Turkey and Coconut Broccoli

Preparation time: 5 minutes **Cooking time**: 25 minutes **Servings:** 4

Ingredients:

1 pound turkey meat, ground 2 garlic cloves, minced

teaspoon ginger, grated

teaspoons coconut aminos 3 tablespoons olive oil

2 broccoli heads, florets separated and then halved A pinch of salt and black pepper

1 teaspoon chili paste

Directions:

Heat up a pan that fits the air fryer with the oil over medium heat, add the meat and brown for 5 minutes. Add the rest of the ingredients, toss, put the pan in the fryer and cook at 380 degrees F for 20 minutes. Divide everything between plates and serve.

Nutrition: calories 274, fat 11, fiber 3, carbs 6, protein 12

Dill Chicken Fritters

Prep time: 20 minutes **Cooking time:** 16 minutes **Servings:** 8

Ingredients:

1-pound chicken breast, skinless, boneless

3 oz coconut flakes

1 tablespoon ricotta cheese

1 teaspoon mascarpone

1 teaspoon dried dill

½ teaspoon salt

1 egg yolk

1 teaspoon avocado oil

Directions:

Cut the chicken breast into the tiny pieces and put them in the bowl. Add coconut flakes, ricotta cheese, mascarpone, dried dill, salt, and egg yolk. Then make the chicken fritters with the help of the fingertips. Preheat the air fryer to 360F. Line the air fryer basket with baking paper and put the chicken cakes in the air fryer. Sprinkle the chicken fritters with avocado oil and cook for 8 minutes. Then flip the chicken fritters on another side and cook them for 8 minutes more.

Nutrition: calories 114, fat 5.9, fiber 1, carbs 1.9, protein 13.1

Turkey and Chili Kale

Preparation time: 5 minutes **Cooking time**: 25 minutes **Servings:** 4

Ingredients:

1 pound turkey meat, ground

A pinch of salt and black pepper 2 tablespoons olive oil

1 teaspoon coconut aminos 2 spring onions, minced

4 cups kale, chopped

1 tablespoon garlic, chopped 1 red chili pepper, chopped

½ cup chicken stock

Directions:

Heat up a pan that fits your air fryer with the oil over medium heat, add the meat, salt, pepper, spring onions and the garlic, stir and sauté for 5 minutes. Add the rest of the ingredients, toss, put the pan in the fryer and cook at 380 degrees F for 20 minutes. Divide between plates and serve

Nutrition: calories 261, fat 12, fiber 2, carbs 5, protein 13

Chili Pepper Duck Bites

Prep time: 15 minutes **Cooking time:** 15 minutes **Servings:** 4

Ingredients:

8 oz duck breast, skinless, boneless

1 teaspoon Erythritol

½ teaspoon salt

1 teaspoon chili pepper

1 tablespoon butter, softened

½ teaspoon minced garlic

½ teaspoon dried dill

Directions:

Cut the duck breast into small pieces (bites). Then sprinkle them with salt, chili pepper, Erythritol, dried dill, and minced garlic. Leave the duck pieces for 10-15 minutes to marinate. Meanwhile, preheat the air fryer to 365F. Sprinkle the duck bites with butter and put in the air fryer. Cook the duck bites for 10 minutes. Then shake them well and cook for 5 minutes more at 400F.

Nutrition: calories 100, fat 5.2, fiber 0.1, carbs 0.3, protein 12.6

Berry Pudding

Preparation time: 5 minutes **Cooking time:** 15 minutes **Servings:** 6

Ingredients:

cups coconut cream 1/3 cup blackberries 1/3 cup blueberries

tablespoons swerve Zest of 1 lime, grated

Directions:

In a blender, combine all the ingredients and pulse well. Divide this into 6 small ramekins, put them in your air fryer and cook at 340 degrees F for 15 minutes. Serve cold.

Nutrition: calories 173, fat 3, fiber 1, carbs 4, protein 4

Butter Crumble

Prep time: 20 minutes **Cooking time:** 25 minutes
Servings: 4

Ingredients:

½ cup coconut flour

2 tablespoons butter, softened

2 tablespoon Erythritol

3 oz peanuts, crushed

1 tablespoon cream cheese

1 teaspoon baking powder

½ teaspoon lemon juice

Directions:

In the mixing bowl mix up coconut flour, butter, Erythritol, baking powder, and lemon juice. Stir the mixture until homogenous. Then place it in the freezer for 10 minutes. Meanwhile, mix up peanuts and cream cheese. Grate the frozen dough. Line the air fryer mold with baking paper. Then put ½ of grated dough in the mold and flatten it. Top it with cream cheese mixture. Then put remaining grated dough over the cream cheese mixture. Place the mold with the crumble in the air fryer and cook it for 25 minutes at 330F.

Nutrition: calories 252, fat 19.6, fiber 7.8, carbs 13.1, protein 8.8

Stevia Cake

Preparation time: 5 minutes **Cooking time:** 40 minutes **Servings:** 6

Ingredients:

2 tablespoons ghee, melted 1 cup coconut, shredded

1 cup mashed avocado 3 tablespoons stevia

teaspoon cinamon powder

2 teaspoons cinnamon powder

Directions:

In a bowl, mix all the ingredients and stir well. Pour this into a cake pan lined with parchment paper, place the pan in the fryer and cook at 340 degrees F for 40 minutes. Cool the cake down, slice and serve.

Nutrition: calories 192, fat 4, fiber 2, carbs 5, protein 7

Sweet Balls

Prep time: 2 **hours Cooking time**: 5 minutes **Servings:** 4

Ingredients:

1 tablespoon cream cheese

3 oz goat cheese

2 tablespoons almond flour

1 tablespoon coconut flour

1 egg, beaten

1 tablespoon Splenda

Cooking spray

Directions:

Mash the goat cheese and mix it up with cream cheese. Then add egg, Splenda, and almond flour. Stir the mixture until homogenous. Then make 4 balls and coat them in the coconut flour. Freeze the cheese balls for 2 hours. Preheat the air fryer to 390F. Then place the frozen balls in the air fryer, spray them with cooking spray and cook for 5 minutes or until the cheese balls are light brown.

Nutrition: calories 224, fat 16.8, fiber 2.3, carbs 7.7, protein 11.4

Chia Cinnamon Pudding

Preparation time: 10 minutes Cooking time: 25 minutes **Servings:** 6

Ingredients:

cups coconut cream 6 egg yolks, whisked 2 tablespoons stevia

¼ cup chia seeds

2 teaspoons cinnamon powder 1 tablespoon ghee, melted

Directions:

In a bowl, mix all the ingredients, whisk, divide into 6 ramekins, place them all in your air fryer and cook at 340 degrees F for 25 minutes. Cool the puddings down and serve.

Nutrition: calories 180, fat 4, fiber 2 carbs 5, protein 7

Seeds and Almond Cookies

Prep time: 15 minutes **Cooking time:** 9 minutes **Servings:** 6

Ingredients:

1 teaspoon chia seeds

1 teaspoon sesame seeds

1 tablespoon pumpkin seeds, crushed

1 egg, beaten

2 tablespoons Splenda

1 teaspoon vanilla extract

1 tablespoon butter

4 tablespoons almond flour

¼ teaspoon ground cloves

1 teaspoon avocado oil

Directions:

Put the chia seeds, sesame seeds, and pumpkin seeds in the bowl. Add egg, Splenda, vanilla extract, butter, avocado oil, and ground cloves. Then add almond flour and mix up the mixture until homogenous. Preheat the air fryer to 375F. Line the air fryer basket with baking paper. With the help of the scooper make the cookies and flatten them gently. Place the cookies in the air fryer. Arrange them in one layer. Cook the seeds cookies for 9 minutes.

Nutrition: calories 180, fat 13.7, fiber 3, carbs 9.6, protein 5.8

Cauliflower Rice Pudding

Preparation time: 5 minutes **Cooking time**: 25 minutes **Servings:** 4

Ingredients:

1 and ½ cups cauliflower rice 2 cups coconut milk

3 tablespoons stevia

2 tablespoons ghee, melted

4 plums, pitted and roughly chopped

Directions:

In a bowl, mix all the ingredients, toss, divide into ramekins, put them in the air fryer, and cook at 340 degrees F for 25 minutes. Cool down and serve.

Nutrition: calories 221, fat 4, fiber 1, carbs 3, protein 3

Peanuts Almond Biscuits

Prep time: 20 minutes **Cooking time:** 35 minutes **Servings:** 6

Ingredients:

4 oz peanuts, chopped

2 tablespoons peanut butter

½ teaspoon apple cider vinegar

1 egg, beaten

6 oz almond flour

¼ cup of coconut milk

2 teaspoons Erythritol

1 teaspoon vanilla extract

Cooking spray

Directions:

In the bowl mix up peanut butter, apple cider vinegar, egg, almond flour, coconut milk, Erythritol, and vanilla extract. When the mixture is homogenous, add peanuts and knead the smooth dough. Then spray the cooking mold with cooking spray and place the dough inside. Preheat the air fryer to 350F. Put the mold with biscuits in the air fryer and cook it for 25 minutes. Then slice the cooked biscuits into pieces and return back in the air fryer. Cook them for 10 minutes more. Cool the cooked biscuits completely.

Nutrition: calories 334, fat 29.1, fiber 5.2, carbs 10.8, protein 13.4

Walnuts and Almonds Granola

Preparation time: 4 minutes **Cooking time**: 8 minutes
Servings: 6

Ingredients:

cup avocado peeled, pitted and cubed

½ cup coconut flakes

tablespoons ghee, melted

¼ cup walnuts, chopped

¼ cup almonds, chopped 2 tablespoons stevia

Directions:

In a pan that fits your air fryer, mix all the ingredients, toss, put the pan in the fryer and cook at 320 degrees F for 8 minutes. Divide into bowls and serve right away.

Nutrition: calories 170, fat 3, fiber 2, carbs 4, protein 3

Hazelnut Vinegar Cookies

Prep time: 25 minutes **Cooking time:** 11 minutes **Servings:** 6

Ingredients:

1 tablespoon flaxseeds

¼ cup flax meal

½ cup coconut flour

½ teaspoon baking powder

1 oz hazelnuts, chopped

1 teaspoon apple cider vinegar

3 tablespoons coconut cream

1 tablespoon butter, softened

3 teaspoons Splenda

Cooking spray

Directions:

Put the flax meal in the bowl. Add flax seeds, coconut flour, baking powder, apple cider vinegar, and Splenda. Stir the mixture gently with the help of the fork and add butter, coconut cream, hazelnuts, and knead the non-sticky dough. If the dough is not sticky enough, add more coconut cream. Make the big ball from the dough and put it in the freezer for 10- 15 minutes. After this, preheat the air fryer to 365F. Make the small balls (cookies) from the flax meal dough and press them gently. Spray the air fryer basket with cooking spray from inside. Arrange the cookies in the air fryer basket in one layer (cook 3-4 cookies per one time) and cook them for 11 minutes. Then transfer the cooked cookies on the plate and cool them completely. Repeat the same steps with remaining uncooked cookies. Store the cookies in the glass jar with the closed lid.

Nutrition: calories 147, fat 10.3, fiber 6.3, carbs 11.1, protein 4.1

Ginger Cod

Prep time: 10 minutes **Cooking time:** 8 minutes **Servings:** 2

Ingredients:

10 oz cod fillet

½ teaspoon cayenne pepper

¼ teaspoon ground coriander

½ teaspoon ground ginger

½ teaspoon ground black pepper

1 tablespoon sunflower oil

½ teaspoon salt

½ teaspoon dried rosemary

½ teaspoon ground paprika

Directions:

In the shallow bowl mix up cayenne pepper, ground coriander, ginger, ground black pepper, salt, dried rosemary, and ground paprika. Then rub the cod fillet with the spice mixture. After this, sprinkle it with sunflower oil. Preheat the air fryer to 390F. Place the cod fillet in the air fryer and cook it for 4 minutes. Then carefully flip the fish on another side and cook for 4 minutes more.

Nutrition: calories 183, fat 8.5, fiber 0.7, carbs 1.4, protein 25.6

Paprika Tilapia

Preparation time: 5 minutes **Cooking time**: 20 minutes **Servings:** 4

Ingredients:

4 tilapia fillets, boneless

3 tablespoons ghee, melted

A pinch of salt and black pepper 2 tablespoons capers

teaspoon garlic powder

½ teaspoon smoked paprika

½ teaspoon oregano, dried 2 tablespoons lemon juice

Directions:

In a bowl, mix all the ingredients except the fish and toss. Arrange the fish in a pan that fits the air fryer, pour the capers mix all over, put the pan in the air fryer and cook 360 degrees F for 20 minutes, shaking halfway.

Divide between plates and serve hot.

Nutrition: calories 224, fat 10, fiber 0, carbs 2, protein 18

Shrimp Skewers

Prep time: 10 minutes **Cooking time:** 5 minutes
Servings: 5

Ingredients:

4-pounds shrimps, peeled

2 tablespoons fresh cilantro, chopped

2 tablespoons apple cider vinegar

1 teaspoon ground coriander

1 tablespoon avocado oil

Cooking spray

Directions:

In the shallow bowl mix up avocado oil, ground coriander, apple cider vinegar, and fresh cilantro. Then put the shrimps in the big bowl and sprinkle with avocado oil mixture. Mix them well and leave for 10 minutes to marinate. After this, string the shrimps on the skewers.

Preheat the air fryer to 400F. Arrange the shrimp skewers in the air fryer and cook them for 5 minutes.

Nutrition: calories 223, fat 14.9, fiber 3.1, carbs 5.5, protein 17.4

Stevia Cod

Preparation time: 5 minutes **Cooking time**: 14 minutes **Servings:** 4

Ingredients:

1/3 cup stevia

tablespoons coconut aminos 4 cod fillets, boneless

A pinch of salt and black pepper

Directions:

In a pan that fits the air fryer, combine all the ingredients and toss gently. Introduce the pan in the fryer and cook at 350 degrees F for 14 minutes, flipping the fish halfway. Divide everything between plates and serve.

Nutrition: calories 267, fat 18, fiber 2, carbs 5, protein 20

Butter Crab Muffins

Prep time: 15 minutes **Cooking time:** 20 minutes **Servings:** 2

Ingredients:

5 oz crab meat, chopped

2 eggs, beaten

2 tablespoons almond flour

¼ teaspoon baking powder

½ teaspoon apple cider vinegar

½ teaspoon ground paprika

1 tablespoon butter, softened

Cooking spray

Directions:

Grind the chopped crab meat and put it in the bowl. Add eggs, almond flour, baking powder, apple cider vinegar, ground paprika, and butter. Stir the mixture until homogenous. Preheat the air fryer to 365F. Spray the muffin molds with cooking spray. Then pour the crab meat batter in the muffin molds and place them in the preheated air fryer. Cook the crab muffins for 20 minutes or until they are light brown. Cool the cooked muffins to the room temperature and remove from the muffin mold.

Nutrition: calories 340, fat 25.5, fiber 3.2, carbs 8.2, protein 20.5

Tilapia and Kale

Preparation time: 5 minutes **Cooking time**: 20 minutes **Servings:** 4

Ingredients:

4 tilapia fillets, boneless

Salt and black pepper to the taste 2 garlic cloves, minced

1 teaspoon fennel seeds

½ teaspoon red pepper flakes, crushed 1 bunch kale, chopped

Table9spoons olive oil

Directions:

In a pan that fits the fryer, combine all the ingredients, put the pan in the fryer and cook at 360 degrees F for 20 minutes. Divide everything between plates and serve.

Nutrition: calories 240, fat 12, fiber 2, carbs 4, protein 12

Chili Haddock

Prep time: 10 minutes **Cooking time:** 8 minutes **Servings:** 4

Ingredients:

12 oz haddock fillet

1 egg, beaten

1 teaspoon cream cheese

1 teaspoon chili flakes

½ teaspoon salt

1 tablespoon flax meal

Cooking spray

Directions:

Cut the haddock on 4 pieces and sprinkle with chili flakes and salt. After this, in the small bowl mix up egg and cream cheese. Dip the haddock pieces in the egg mixture and generously sprinkle with flax meal. Preheat the air fryer to 400F. Put the prepared haddock pieces in the air fryer in one layer and cook them for 4 minutes from each side or until they are golden brown.

Nutrition: calories 122, fat 2.8, fiber 0.5, carbs 0.6, protein 22.5

Lime Cod

Preparation time: 5 minutes **Cooking time**: 14 minutes **Servings:** 4

Ingredients:

cod fillets, boneless 1 tablespoon olive oil

Salt and black pepper to the taste 2 teaspoons sweet paprika

Juice of 1 lime

Directions:

In a bowl, mix all the ingredients, transfer the fish to your air fryer's basket and cook 350 degrees F for 7 minutes on each side. Divide the fish between plates and serve with a side salad.

Nutrition: calories 240, fat 14, fiber 2, carbs 4, protein 16

Mackerel with Spring Onions and Peppers

Prep time: 15 minutes **Cooking time:** 20 minutes **Servings:** 5

Ingredients:

1-pound mackerel, trimmed

1 tablespoon ground paprika

1 green bell pepper

½ cup spring onions, chopped

1 tablespoon avocado oil

1 teaspoon apple cider vinegar

½ teaspoon salt

Directions:

Wash the mackerel if needed and sprinkle with ground paprika. Chop the green bell pepper. Then fill the mackerel with bell pepper and spring onion. After this, sprinkle the fish with avocado oil, apple cider vinegar, and salt. Preheat the air fryer to 375F. Place the mackerel in the air fryer basket and cook it for 20 minutes.

Nutrition: calories 258, fat 16.8, fiber 1.2, carbs 3.8, protein 22.2

Ginger Salmon

Preparation time: 5 minutes **Cooking time**: 12 minutes **Servings:** 4

Ingredients:

2 tablespoons lime juice

1 pound salmon fillets, boneless, skinless and cubed 1 tablespoon ginger, grated

4 teaspoons olive oil

1 tablespoon coconut aminos

1 tablespoon sesame seeds, toasted 1 tablespoon chives, chopped

Directions:

In a pan that fits the air fryer, combine all the ingredients, toss, introduce in the fryer and cook at 360 degrees F for 12 minutes. Divide into bowls and serve.

Nutrition: calories 206, fat 8, fiber 1, carbs 4, protein 13

Cheesy Sausage Sticks

Prep time: 15 minutes **Cooking time:** 8 minutes
Servings: 3

Ingredients:

6 small pork sausages

½ cup almond flour

½ cup Mozzarella cheese, shredded

2 eggs, beaten

1 tablespoon mascarpone

Cooking spray

Directions:

Pierce the hot dogs with wooden coffee sticks to get the sausages on the sticks". Then in the bowl mix up almond flour, Mozzarella cheese, and mascarpone. Microwave the mixture for 15 seconds or until you get a melted mixture. Then stir the egg in the cheese mixture and whisk it until smooth. Coat every sausage stick in the cheese mixture. Then preheat the air fryer to 375F. Spray the air fryer basket with cooking spray. Place the sausage stock in the air fryer and cook them for 4 minutes from each side or until they are light brown.

Nutrition: calories 375, fat 32.2, fiber 0.5, carbs 5.1, protein 16.3

Avocado and Cabbage Salad

Preparation time: 5 minutes **Cooking time**: 15 minutes **Servings:** 4

Ingredients:

cups red cabbage, shredded A drizzle of olive oil

1 red bell pepper, sliced

small avocado, peeled, pitted and sliced Salt and black pepper to the taste

Directions:

Grease your air fryer with the oil, add all the ingredients, toss, cover and cook at 400 degrees F for 15 minutes. Divide into bowls and serve cold for breakfast.

Nutrition: calories 209, fat 8, fiber 2, carbs 4, protein 9

Lemon and Almond Cookies

Prep time: 10 minutes **Cooking time:** 8 minutes **Servings:** 4

Ingredients:

4 tablespoons coconut flour

½ teaspoon baking powder

1 teaspoon lemon juice

¼ teaspoon vanilla extract

¼ teaspoon lemon zest, grated

2 eggs, beaten

¼ cup of organic almond milk

1 teaspoon avocado oil

¼ teaspoon Himalayan pink salt

Directions:

In the big bowl mix up all ingredients from the list above. Knead the soft dough and cut it into 4 pieces. Preheat the air fryer to 400F. Then line the air fryer basket with baking paper. Roll the dough pieces in the balls and press them gently to get the shape of flat cookies. Place the cookies in the air fryer and cook them for 8 minutes.

Nutrition: calories 74, fat 3.8, fiber 3.1, carbs 5.6, protein 4.4

Mushroom Bake

Preparation time: 5 minutes **Cooking time**: 20 minutes **Servings:** 4

Ingredients:

garlic cloves, minced 1 teaspoon olive oil

2 celery stalks, chopped

½ cup white mushrooms, chopped

½ cup red bell pepper, chopped Salt and black pepper to the taste 1 teaspoon oregano, dried

7 ounces mozzarella, shredded 1 tablespoon lemon juice

Directions:

Preheat the Air Fryer at 350 degrees F, add the oil and heat it up. Add garlic, celery, mushrooms, bell pepper, salt, pepper, oregano, mozzarella and the lemon juice, toss and cook for 20 minutes. Divide between plates and serve for breakfast.

Nutrition: calories 230, fat 11, fiber 2, carbs 4, protein 6

Spiced Cauliflower and Ham Quiche

Prep time: 10 minutes **Cooking time:** 15 minutes **Servings:** 4

Ingredients:

5 eggs, beaten

½ cup heavy cream

1 teaspoon ground nutmeg

¼ teaspoon ground cardamom

¼ teaspoon salt

1 teaspoon ground black pepper

1 teaspoon butter, softened

¼ cup spring onions, chopped

¼ cup cauliflower florets

5 oz ham, chopped

3 oz Provolone cheese, grated

Directions:

Pour the beaten eggs in the bowl. Add heavy cream, ground nutmeg, ground cardamom, ground black pepper, and salt. After this, pour the liquid in the air fryer round pan. Add butter, onion, cauliflower florets, ham, and cheese. Gently stir the quiche liquid. Place it in the air fryer and cook the quiche for 15 minutes at 385F.

Nutrition: calories 280, fat 20.9, fiber 1.1, carbs 4.4, protein 18.9

Spiced Pudding

Preparation time: 4 **minutes Cooking time**: 12 minutes **Servings:** 2

Ingredients:

½ teaspoon cinnamon powder

¼ teaspoon allspice, ground 4 tablespoons erythritol

4 eggs, whisked

2 tablespoons heavy cream Cooking spray

Directions:

In a bowl, mix all the ingredients except the cooking spray, whisk well and pour into a ramekin greased with cooking spray. Add the basket to your Air Fryer, put the ramekin inside and cook at 400 degrees F for 12 minutes. Divide into bowls and serve for breakfast.

Nutrition: calories 201, fat 11, fiber 2, carbs 4, protein 6

Bacon Pockets

Prep time: 15 minutes **Cooking time:** 4 minutes
Servings: 6

Ingredients:

6 wontons wrap

1 egg yolk, whisked

2 oz bacon, chopped, cooked

½ cup Edam cheese, shredded

1 teaspoon sesame oil

½ teaspoon ground black pepper

Directions:

Put the chopped bacon in the bowl. Add Edam cheese and ground black pepper. Stir the ingredients gently with the help of the fork. After this, put the mixture on the wonton wrap and fold it in the shape of the pocket.

Repeat the steps with remaining filling and wonton wraps. Preheat the air fryer to 400F. Brush every wonton pocket with whisked egg yolk. Then brush the air fryer with sesame oil and arrange the pockets inside. Cook the meal for 2 minutes from each side.

Nutrition: calories 136, fat 10.1, fiber 0.1, carbs 2.6, protein 8.6

Green Beans and Eggs

Preparation time: 5 minutes **Cooking time:** 20 minutes **Servings:** 4

Ingredients:

pound green beans, roughly chopped Cooking spray

eggs, whisked

Salt and black pepper to the taste 1 tablespoon sweet paprika

ounces sour cream

Directions:

Grease a pan that fits your air fryer with the cooking spray and mix all the ingredients inside. Put the pan in the Air Fryer and cook at 360 degrees F for 20 minutes. Divide between plates and serve.

Nutrition: calories 220, fat 14, fiber 2, carbs 3, protein 2

Basil Tomato Bowls

Preparation time: 5 minutes **Cooking time**: 15 minutes **Servings:** 4

Ingredients:

1 pound cherry tomatoes, halved 1 cup mozzarella, shredded Cooking spray

Salt and black pepper to the taste 1 teaspoon basil, chopped

Directions:

Grease the tomatoes with the cooking spray, season with salt and pepper, sprinkle the mozzarella on top, place them all in your air fryer's basket, cook at 330 degrees F for 15 minutes, divide into bowls, sprinkle the basil on top and serve.

Nutrition: calories 140, fat 7, fiber 3, carbs 4, protein 5

Tofu Wraps

Prep time: 15 minutes **Cooking time:** 9 minutes **Servings:** 4

Ingredients:

4 low carb tortillas

5 oz tofu, cubed

1 teaspoon mustard

1 teaspoon avocado oil

1 teaspoon lemon juice

½ cup white cabbage, shredded

4 teaspoons cream cheese

2 chipotles, chopped

Directions:

Preheat the air fryer to 400F. Meanwhile, mix up mustard with avocado oil and lemon juice. Place the tofu cubes in the mustard mixture and coat them well. Then put the tofu in the air fryer basket and cook for 9 minutes. Shake the tofu during cooking for 2-3 times to avoid burning. Then place the tofu on the tortillas. Add shredded cabbage, chipotles, and cream cheese. Fold the wraps.

Nutrition: calories 133, fat 5.1, fiber 8.1, carbs 15.7, protein 6.9

Sage Cream

Preparation time: 5 minutes **Cooking time**: **30 minutes Servings:** 4

Ingredients:

7 cups red currants 1 cup swerve

1 cup water

6 sage leaves

Directions:

In a pan that fits your air fryer, mix all the ingredients, toss, put the pan in the fryer and cook at 330 degrees F for 30 minutes. Discard sage leaves, divide into cups and serve cold.

Nutrition: calories 171, fat 4, fiber 2, carbs 3, protein 6

Peanut Butter Cookies

Prep time: 30 minutes **Cooking time:** 20 minutes **Servings:** 4

Ingredients:

½ cup almond flour

2 tablespoons butter, softened

1 tablespoon Splenda

¼ teaspoon vanilla extract

4 teaspoons peanut butter

1 teaspoon Erythritol

Cooking spray

Directions:

Make the cookies: put the almond flour and butter in the bowl. Add Splenda and vanilla extract and knead the non-sticky dough. Then cut dough on 8 pieces. Make the balls and press them to get the flat cookies. Preheat the air fryer to 365F. Spray the air fryer basket with cooking spray and put the cookies in the air fryer in one layer – make 4 flat cookies per one time). Cook them for 10 minutes. Repeat the same steps with remaining cookies. Cool the cooked flat cookies completely. Meanwhile, mix up Erythritol and peanut butter. Then spread 4 flat cookies with peanut butter mixture and cover them with remaining cookies.

Nutrition: calories 118, fat 10.2, fiber 0.7, carbs 4.8, protein 2.1

Currant Cream Ramekins

Preparation time: 5 minutes **Cooking time**: 20 minutes **Servings:** 6

Ingredients:

1 cup red currants, blended

1 cup black currants, blended 3 tablespoons stevia

cup coconut cream

Directions:

In a bowl, combine all the ingredients and stir well. Divide into ramekins, put them in the fryer and cook at 340 degrees F for 20 minutes. Serve the pudding cold.

Nutrition: calories 200, fat 4, fiber 2, carbs 4, protein 6

Clove Crackers

Prep time: 20 minutes **Cooking time:** 33 minutes **Servings:** 8

Ingredients:

1 cup almond flour

1 teaspoon xanthan gum

1 teaspoon flax meal

½ teaspoon salt

1 teaspoon baking powder

1 teaspoon lemon juice

½ teaspoon ground clove

2 tablespoons Erythritol

1 egg, beaten

3 tablespoons coconut oil, softened

Directions:

In the mixing bowl mix up almond flour, xanthan gum, flax meal, salt, baking powder, and ground clove. Add Erythritol, lemon juice, egg, and coconut oil. Stir the mixture gently with the help of the fork. Then knead the mixture till you get a soft dough. Line the chopping board with parchment. Put the dough on the parchment and roll it up in a thin layer. Cut the thin dough into squares (crackers). Preheat the air fryer to 360F. Line the air fryer basket with baking paper. Put the prepared crackers in the air fryer basket in one layer and cook them for 11 minutes or until the crackers are dry and light brown. Repeat the same steps with remaining uncooked crackers.

Nutrition: calories 79, fat 7.5, fiber 1.8, carbs 2.5, protein 1.5

Currant Vanilla Cookies

Preparation time: 5 minutes **Cooking time**: 30 minutes **Servings**: 6

Ingredients:

cups almond flour

2 teaspoons baking soda

½ cup ghee, melted

½ cup swerve

1 teaspoon vanilla extract

½ cup currants

Directions:

In a bowl, mix all the ingredients and whisk well. Spread this on a baking sheet lined with parchment paper, put the pan in the air fryer and cook at 350 degrees F for 30 minutes. Cool down, cut into rectangles and serve.

Nutrition: calories 172, fat 5, fiber 2, carbs 3, protein 5

Chocolate Fudge

Prep time: 15 minutes **Cooking time:** 30 minutes **Servings:** 8

Ingredients:

½ cup butter, melted

1 oz dark chocolate, chopped, melted

2 tablespoons cocoa powder

3 tablespoons coconut flour

1 teaspoon vanilla extract

2 eggs, beaten

3 tablespoons Splenda

Cooking spray

Directions:

In the bowl mix up melted butter and dark chocolate. Then add vanilla extract, eggs, and cocoa powder. Stir the mixture until smooth and add Splenda, and coconut flour. Stir it again until smooth. Then preheat the air fryer to 325F. Line the air fryer basket with baking paper and spray it with cooking spray. Pour the fudge mixture in the air fryer basket, flatten it gently with the help of the spatula. Cook the fudge for 30 minutes. Then cut it on the serving squares and cool the fudge completely.

Nutrition: calories 177, fat 14.8, fiber 1.6, carbs 8.3, protein 2.6

Cranberries Pudding

Preparation time: 5 minutes **Cooking time**: 20 minutes **Servings:** 6

Ingredients:

1 cup cauliflower rice 2 cups almond milk

½ cup cranberries

1 teaspoon vanilla extract

Directions:

In a pan that fits your air fryer, mix all the ingredients, whisk a bit, put the pan in the fryer and cook at 360 degrees F for 20 minutes. Stir the pudding, divide into bowls and serve cold.

Nutrition: calories 211, fat 5, fiber 2, carbs 4, protein 7

Merengues

Prep time: 15 minutes **Cooking time:** 65 minutes
Servings: 6

Ingredients:

2 egg whites

1 teaspoon lime zest, grated

1 teaspoon lime juice

4 tablespcons Erythritol

Directions:

Whisk the egg whites until soft peaks. Then add Erythritol
and lime juice and whisk the egg whites until you get
strong peaks. After this, add lime zest and carefully stir
the egg white mixture. Preheat the air fryer to 275F. Line
the air fryer basket with baking paper. With the help of
the spoon make the small merengues and put them in
the air fryer in one layer. Cook the dessert for 65
minutes.

Nutrition: calories 6, fat 0, fiber 0, carbs 0.2, protein 1.2

Lemon Coconut Bars

Preparation time: 10 minutes **Cooking time:** 20 minutes **Servings:** 12

Ingredients:

1 cup coconut cream

¼ cup cashew butter, soft

¾ cup swerve 1 egg, whisked

Juice of 1 lemon

1 teaspoon lemon peel, grated 1 teaspoon baking powder

Directions:

In a bowl, combine all the ingredients gradually and stir well. Spoon balls this on a baking sheet lined with parchment paper and flatten them. Put the sheet in the fryer and cook at 350 degrees F for 20 minutes. Cut into bars and serve cold.

Nutrition: calories 121, fat 5, fiber 1, carbs 4, protein 2

Lightning Source UK Ltd.
Milton Keynes UK
UKHW052314291022
411228UK00013B/106

9 781803 423784